Self Healing 101

How to Emotionally Heal Yourself and
Methodically Solve your Problems
without the Use of Traditional Therapy

By Blaine Williams

Table of Contents

Introduction

It is not always necessary to pay lots of money to see some swanky therapist. You may not be able to afford traditional therapy, you may not have time, or you may not find that lying on a couch and talking about your problems to a clinically trained stranger is helpful in any way. Regardless of why you do not want to use traditional therapeutic approaches to your problems, you can forego traditional therapy and heal yourself using a variety of emotional self-healing methods.

Self-healing is certainly possible. You really can balm your emotional wounds, correct your harmful thinking habits, and balance your emotions without the help of a trained therapist. The power to become well emotionally and mentally lies within you. You just have to unlock this power. There are a variety of self-healing approaches that you can use to unlock your self-healing power and become well again. This book contains some of the main approaches that you may have great luck with while healing yourself.

Self-healing is not an easy task. In fact, it may be one of the most difficult things that you ever accomplish. However, it is certainly worth the effort. There are so many benefits to using self-healing. By healing your wounds, you no longer suffer in life. You also prove to yourself that you are strong and capable. You will improve your thinking and self-love and gain great habits that will help prevent you from further emotional harm in the future. Finally, you can learn from your mistakes and your failures and avoid committing the same things in the future. After using self-healing, you will gain a better understanding of yourself and you will emerge from the journey as an improved version of yourself.

Just be prepared for a lot of hard work. Also be prepared for some setbacks and backslides. It will not all be smooth sailing. However, using the methods of self-healing discussed in this book will ensure that you are successful. You will be much better off after you employ these methods on yourself.

Good luck on your self-healing journey. Start transforming yourself and closing your emotional wounds today. There is no point to waiting.

Chapter 1: Basic Principles of Self-Healing

Self-healing is a basic function of your consciousness. Emotional wounds are an inevitable part of life. During at least one part of your life, you will probably experience a rejection or a tragedy which will hurt you deeply. This traumatic event will make you question yourself and your inner abilities. It will also make you question life and its fairness. Being able to heal is therefore a necessary facet of life that your subconscious mind is naturally equipped for. But activating this self-healing ability can take some effort, especially if you have experienced multiple emotional wounds that have left you feeling incomplete and incapable of healing.

Here are some basic concepts of self-healing that you must understand before embarking on the self-healing journey. Understanding these concepts can help you develop the attitude that you need to begin the process. You can change your lifestyle and your thinking to facilitate self-healing as a natural internal process. You can also cut out things that are prone to interfering with your healing.

Have a Goal

Humans are goal-oriented. This means that having a goal is very necessary to your self-healing. By having a specific goal in mind, you teach your mind what it should focus on. You open yourself up to a specific emotional wound that you need to address.

The goals that you set for self-healing are entirely up to you. Analyze what causes you the most pain and focus on those things first. You might want to grow your self-esteem and your confidence, for instance. You might want to improve your ability to let go of past grievances and move on with life. You might want to learn to forgive, and work on forgiving a certain person that caused you a lot of pain. Perhaps there is a specific trauma in your past that you want to work on getting over. You may also want to improve your thinking, so that you become a more positive and happy person overall. You know in your heart what goals you should make for your self-healing.

Take Control

Like most people, you probably don't realize the sheer level of control that you really do exert over yourself. You may feel that you live at the mercy of your emotions and your body, but this is because you do not exert your power over yourself. You let your emotions run unchecked. However, you need to realize that you actually have complete control. If you so desire, you can check your emotions and your body so that you have total control.

As part of self-healing, you need to fully actualize your control over yourself. Stop living at the mercy of your emotions, and instead fearlessly take charge. Kick out bad emotions and cultivate positive ones. Give your body and mind specific orders in an authoritative tone and then make your body and mind obey. This may seem impossible, but it is not. Once you start taking control, you will be surprised at how easily you can access your emotions and make yourself behave as you wish.

You can order yourself to feel better and have more energy. You can also order yourself to stop obsessing over your ex or your abusive family members. Whatever you want your mind to do is entirely possible.

Love Yourself

One of the most basic yet most important premises of self-healing is self-love. How can you possibly heal yourself if you are constantly hurting yourself with self-loathing? The mean things that you think about yourself are really just chipping away at your self-esteem, thought by thought. You are making it very hard to heal when you are doing lots of damage to yourself. In addition, you can't heal yourself if you don't love yourself because you will not believe that you are worthy of feeling better and being happy. Your attitude alone sabotages your self-healing process.

Therefore, you must get into the habit of practicing self-love. Treat yourself with dignity and respect. Speak to yourself nicely. Focus more on your accomplishments, talents, and positive attributes than your failures, flaws, and lacks. In the long run, you will start treating yourself better and you will open the doors to self-healing. You will also begin to feel better and enjoy life more, as you remove the negative self-loathing that hurts you so much.

Self-love is really just a habit. Like all good habits, it will take time to cultivate it. You may be caught in the habit of self-loathing, as many people are. Just be patient with yourself. When you catch yourself thinking mean things about yourself, just divert your thoughts up more positive and loving channels. Don't beat yourself up just because you have a tough time loving yourself at first.

One thing that helps is imagining yourself as a small child. You are a cute kid, new to the world. Take delight in your infant self, just as you would take delight in seeing a baby in real life. Coddle yourself, just as you would a baby. You are that baby. You will slowly get into the habit of thinking of yourself with the same love and tenderness as you would think of an adorable newborn.

Positive Thinking

Each thought that you think triggers a corresponding emotion, whether you realize it or not. If you think mostly negative thoughts, then it is a small wonder why your moods are mostly negative. You will suffer from depression, anxiety, and unhappiness as a result of your negative thinking. You can eliminate this problem by adjusting your thinking to be more positive. Positive thinking will end up boosting your mood and giving you joy, hope, motivation, and enthusiasm.

It may take some time to get into the habit of thinking positively. That is OK. Be patient with yourself and count the effort that you must put into changing your thinking habits as an essential part of the self-healing process. In the end, you will have more control over your thoughts and you will also feel much better. You can effectively eliminate depression and misery from your life just by becoming more positive in your thinking processes. Whenever you think something negative, chase it with a more positive thought. Also try to think positively right off the bat.

Positive thinking isn't being happy about everything all of the time. That is an unrealistic expectation. Rather, positive thinking takes negative experiences and finds the good in them. It also seeks to find reasonable, helpful solutions to your problems. You get into the habit of thinking nice things about yourself and thinking of how grateful you are for certain things in your life. Instead of fixating on the negative things in your life, you choose to fixate on the positive. You become focused on the good in life, as well as the good within yourself. You also become more enthusiastic for living and for the challenges that life represents.

Believe that You can Get Well

What you believe has a major impact on what your mind feels that it can achieve. You will not get well if you do not believe that you will. You must believe in your ability to heal in order to convince your mind that self-healing is possible and not a huge waste of time. Your mind will only comply with what it views as possible. Therefore, make your mind comply with self-healing by believing that your self-healing efforts will work and that your attempts to heal your internal wounds are not in vain.

Dedication and Focus

Self-healing takes dedication and focus. You must dedicate time and effort to self-healing. You must be willing to exhaust all measures to heal yourself, while never giving up. Self-healing must be a priority that you put first in life. After all, you can only overcome your issues once you start healing them, so make self-healing number one in your life.

It is important to understand that self-healing is an active process. It requires your involvement. You must be prepared to dedicating some serious time and effort to healing yourself. The process will not happen overnight and it will not be handed to you. Rather, it is an undertaking that you must commit to. Be prepared to dedicate some of your strength and time to this undertaking.

Focus on healing, not on your problems or your mental health issues. By focusing on the positive rather than the negative, you will encourage yourself to make forward progress. You will not encourage your disease or problems by fixating on them. The things in your life that you give attention will grow, so avoid growing your problems and instead grow your healing power and happiness.

Healthy Lifestyle

You cannot reasonably expect to heal yourself if you are busy harming yourself with an unhealthy lifestyle. Your lifestyle has a direct effect on how well you feel. Your mental processes and physical health are tied together, so you want to stimulate and support both your mental and physical well-being in the way that you choose to live.

To feel better, you must have a healthy lifestyle. You must eat well and nourish your body. This in turn will nourish your mind. Often, mental sluggishness and depression is related to deficiencies in the vitamins and minerals in your body. Therefore, a healthy diet and good supplements will help support both your mental and physical health.

Exercise also reduces stress and helps you feel better. As you get fitter, you become more confident about your body, as well. Therefore, you should try to fit exercise into your routine. Try to get at least twenty minutes of cardio in at least three times a week. Conditioning, such as yoga or Tai Chi, is also great for your stress reduction and overall wellness.

Finally, cut out the bad things in life. These include stressful friends, tense situations, and unhealthy activities such as drinking or smoking. You are only subjecting yourself to harm and inhibiting your healing process with these activities. You want to surround yourself with health and positivity, so cut out the things that reduce your happiness and health and safety. Stop talking to negative friends and avoid the habits that hurt you. You can only prosper if you have a lifestyle that encourages prosperity and gives you room for growth.

View your Setbacks and Problems as Lessons

Part of becoming more positive involves changing your attitude about the bad things that have happened to you. You can change your attitude to be more positive about bad things in your past. "How can I do this?" you may ask yourself. Some things in life may seem too horrible to ever be positive about. Well, you can do this by viewing each bad thing, each setback, and each failure as an opportunity for learning and growth. Each terrible thing in your past is a lesson that you can use to make your future and present better.

When you attempt to learn from the bad things in your life, you add a level of positivity to these things. You make the bad things in your life have a purpose. You reap these bad things for every ounce of good that they can possibly offer you. This offers you a certain degree of peace, as you begin to view bad events and failures in a more positive light. You change your relationship with the difficulties in life, from one of a despair and misery to one of growth and positivity.

Each bad event in your life actually offers you a great deal of potential benefit. You can really use these events to grow. By looking at the bad things in life from this perspective, you encourage yourself to think of how you could do things differently in the future. Instead of drowning in the misery that regret and hindsight can bring you, however, you let yourself become excited at how you can make your future better. You really will learn a lot and grow as a person. You will help make your future much easier as you let the lessons of your past help you.

In addition, you learn to become more resilient in the future. When something bad happens, you stop beating yourself up. Instead, you focus on how to use the experience for your personal growth. You start to take a more problem-solving and introspective approach to the bad things in your life, rather than a useless and overly emotional approach.

Stay in the Present

I will discuss this topic in more depth in the section on mindfulness. However, I must touch on it here because staying in the present moment is absolutely essential to your self-healing. Being focused on what is currently going on in your present moment really helps you gain control over your thoughts and emotions. It also helps you conserve your energy, so that you invest it in healing. By not worrying about the past or the future, you reduce your stress and anxiety levels. There are numerous benefits to reining in your thoughts and staying in the current moment, so be sure to practice mindfulness. Read on for more about this fascinating and helpful topic in Chapter 3.

Accept Setbacks as Part of the Healing Process

The healing process is a long and sometimes difficult one. You will not always meet your goals. You will not always make forward progress. Some days will just be tough, and there is really nothing that you can do about that.

Narcotics Anonymous encourages drug addicts to accept relapse as a natural and very possible part of the healing process. Often, addicts will experience relapses. These relapses do not mean that the healing is over. An addict can have a relapse and then continue working toward sobriety. Narcotics Anonymous strives to make it clear that a relapse does not mean that you have failed in healing.

This same principle applies to all other aspects of self-healing. If you are trying to recover from depression or an eating disorder, for instance, you may be doing well. Then one day you just become depressed or you feel fat and you force yourself to throw up after a meal. You may feel that this relapse means that you have failed at your attempt to heal, but just as with people recovering from addiction, relapse is really just a part of the healing process. It is almost inevitable. Do not beat yourself up over a relapse.

Instead, use the misery that a relapse causes you as a reminder why you started self-healing in the first place. Let it strengthen your resolve. Press on without giving up. Do not let a relapse derail your progress in healing. Once a relapse is over, you can continue with your healing journey. It is not over yet!

One way to minimize the pain and disappointment of a relapse is to remind yourself that you are not perfect. Accept that a relapse may occur. That way, when it does occur, you will not feel so shocked, angry, and disappointed. You should also have a backup plan for when you do relapse. Determine what steps to take to resume your healing journey and recover from the relapse with minimal pain and damage to yourself. Decide early on not to beat yourself up over a relapse, either. Practice lots of self-love and self-forgiveness in these events.

Add Joy to Your Life

When you are completely miserable, you may blame that misery on your extenuating life circumstances. You may think that your life is just not permitting you to enjoy yourself and be happy. However, keep in mind that your happiness is really an attitude and a state of mind that you practice. Life will never calm down and hand you happiness; you must eke it out for yourself.

One of the best ways to improve your happiness is to add as much joy as you can to your life. Even with your extenuating circumstances, you can at least add a few minutes of happiness to your days. Stop using your unhappy situation or your life problems as excuses to ignore the opportunities for joy, laughter, and love. Just a few minutes of joy can really make a huge difference on how you feel, especially if the rest of your life seems bleak.

How can you add joy to your life? There are many ways. You could do a craft or hobby that you love. You could volunteer somewhere so that you make good friends and feel useful as you see the meaningful impact you have on others. You could go on a day trip somewhere. You could spend time laughing with your family, perhaps playing a board game or even just eating a good home-cooked meal together. Even just watching your favorite movie, getting your nails manicured, or going for a walk can bring you significant joy and can take your mind off of whatever is bothering you. Whatever brings you joy should be a staple in your daily life.

Chapter 2: Cognitive Behavioral Therapy

Cognitive behavioral therapy, hereafter referred to CBT, targets your negative thinking habits and attempts to change them into more positive ones. You can end the harmful ways that you think and instead teach yourself to think along more helpful lines with CBT. The great thing about CBT is that you can use it on yourself. You just need to download a free CBT workbook online or keep a journal.

CBT believes that your pain and suffering arises when you think along certain bad lines, known as cognitive distortions. You essentially distort your life in a negative way. Once you isolate the cognitive distortions that you have, you can start to affect changes and think along more helpful paths. You can work through negative events in your life that cause you pain by thinking about them in more positive, helpful ways.

Cognitive Distortions

When you distort something in your life, you cause yourself a lot of pain. Here are the main cognitive distortions. You will probably recognize some of them, as they are very common patterns of unhelpful thinking.

- **Filtering** – You focus too much on the negative. You filter out all of the positive aspects of a situation. Try looking for positive aspects to every situation instead of fixating on the negative.

- **Black and White Thinking –** You believe that everything is sunshine and rainbows or horrible and morbid. Nothing is ever in a gray area. Try seeing how things are balanced between good and bad. This is a far more realistic form of thinking.

- **Overgeneralization –** You assume that bad things will happen over and over. You always expect the same outcome for every situation, just because something bad happened to you once in the past. For instance, if your ex cheated on you, you might think that all men or women are cheaters and that you will always be cheated on by everyone that you date.

- **Jumping to Conclusions** – You assume what someone is thinking or feeling. You read meaning into what someone says without asking. You often draw conclusions on your own with no basis for these conclusions. As a result, you may cause yourself a lot of pain by assuming that something is true when it is not. Try not to do this. Instead, seek information before drawing a conclusion. Also learn to be flexible and to consider that your conclusions about situations may be incorrect. Adjust your conclusions with evidence.

- **Catastrophizing** – You feel that you are on the brink of disaster at any time. Fear riddles your life. If someone doesn't call, you work yourself into a panic thinking that he or she is dead. Stop always expecting the very worse. Usually things are just fine.

- **Personalization** – You think that everything is about you. You blame yourself for things that you have no control over. In addition, you think that everything people say or do is a direct personal attack on you. Remember that most people think about things other than you and you are not the center of the universe for everyone.

- **Control Fallacies** – You believe that you are somehow in control and responsible for everyone's fate if you suffer from an internal control fallacy. On the other hand, if you have an external control fallacy, you believe that you are helpless at the hands of fate and you blame everyone and everything else for your problems or mistakes. Realize that you are neither helpless nor responsible for everything in the world.

- **Fallacy of Fairness** – You believe that you know what is fair. Therefore, when your idea of fairness is not met, you become bitter and resentful. Remember that you really do not know what is fair and your beliefs about what is fair have nothing to do with life or how life works. Life could not care less about your idea of fair.

- **Blaming** – You have to find someone or something to blame for everything. You may blame yourself or you may blame others, but either way you get incredibly frustrated and angry with the object of your blame. Understand that some things are no one's fault and that blame does not fix problems. Focus more on fixing problems rather than finding a source of fault.

- **Should Thinking** – Your life is ruled by certain rigid ideas that you hold. You think you know how things should be, and you are very disappointed when life does not work as it "should." You set yourself up for disappointment by holding this cognitive distortion, so avoid thinking about how things should be.

- **Emotional Reasoning** – You reason based on your emotions and falsely assume that everything that you feel is true. You may believe that you are boring, for instance, because you feel boring. But know that emotions are not always accurate indicators of reality.

- **Fallacy of Change** – You believe that you can change others into what you want. You give yourself a false sense of importance and you believe that your happiness is based on the behavior of others. When people refuse to change, you find yourself very hurt. People cannot be changed so don't try.

- **Global Labeling** – You meet one person from a race who is rude, so you assume that the entire race is rude. You make global judgements based on inadequate evidence, thus narrowing your view of the world in an unhealthy and unhelpful way. You need to gather more evidence before making any kind of generalization, and you should be prepared for your generalization to be wrong.

- **Always Being Right** – Being right is so important to you that you will do anything to prove your rightness. In truth, you may be wrong, or you may be right but someone will never accept that. Give up the fight because being right is not the most important thing in the entire world.

- **Heaven's Reward Fallacy** – You believe that you are owed some sort of reward for being a good person. Therefore, you are bitter when the reward never comes. Don't expect to be rewarded for being a good person. The world doesn't appreciate goodness. Just appreciate yourself and move on.

How to Use CBT

To begin using CBT on yourself to fix your thinking, you should start a CBT journal. Document your progress. This journal will be very helpful in organizing your thoughts and documenting the progress that you make.

Identify Cognitive Distortions

You must comb your thinking to identify cognitive distortions. When you encounter an event that upsets you, write it down in your journal. Then go through your thoughts about the event. Are you using any cognitive distortions? If so, what are they? Be sure to write them down. Also document how each cognitive distortion makes you feel and how you feel about the event overall.

Find More Helpful Thinking

For every cognitive distortion that you identify in your thinking about an event, there is a more positive alternative. Write down better, more helpful ways that you could think about the event. As a result, you will find that you feel better about the event. Write down how you feel now and you will notice that you have brought about a positive change in both your thinking and your emotions. Your thoughts directly influence your emotions, so changing your thinking patterns can help you feel much better.

In your day-to-day life, thinking in more positive ways will become habit. You will start to see when you are thinking with a cognitive distortion and you will know how to change your thinking to be more helpful and uplifting.

Become Solution-Oriented

When you are faced with a problem in life, don't just drown in negative emotions. Instead, dedicate your focus and energy on solving your problems in a satisfactory manner. Use your journal to help you brainstorm solutions to your problems. Often, solutions lie just in changing

your thinking.

Chapter 3: Mindfulness

A recent Harvard study found that people who have wandering minds are more prone to unhappiness than people who stay mindful of the present moment. People who are able to focus on the present are able to ground their minds and control their thoughts. Therefore, they are better able to keep cheerful attitudes and slash issues such as depression.

Achieving mindfulness helps ground you in your present. It allows you to become more aware of your thoughts, so that you can cut out negative thoughts that are detrimental to your happiness. By making mindfulness a habit in your lifestyle, you can become a happier person. Consider mindfulness a mental exercise that can really help you heal yourself by allowing you to control your thinking and get rid of harmful thinking patterns.

How to Achieve Mindfulness

Mindfulness is simply a form of awareness. You can teach yourself to be more mindful with practice and dedication. Keep in mind that this is a mental exercise that calls for discipline. You will not become totally mindful after one day. In time, however, you can adjust your mind to be mindful at all times.

Start practicing mindfulness in little increments. Clear some time and space for yourself. Sit still. Focus on the feeling of your breath coming in through your nostrils and going out through your mouth. Count your breaths and really focus on the way your body feels as the air fills your lungs. When thoughts try to intrude, gently ignore them and turn your attention back to your breathing. Slowly go through each muscle in your body, tightening then relaxing each body part. It is easiest to start with your right-hand thumb, move up your arm to your shoulder and neck, go down the right side of your body to your toes, then move to your left toes and go all the way till you reach your left-hand thumb. Paying attention to your muscles and your breath so resolutely will help anchor your mind to the present and banish unwanted thoughts.

Also, when you are engaged in a task, try to practice becoming totally mindful of that task. For instance, if you are washing dishes, fixate on the sound of the sponge wiping the glass. Really focus on the sensation of the soap suds on your hands. If you are wearing gloves, focus on how the rubber feels on your skin. Just be totally in the moment. Another example is when you are driving. Usually your mind drifts while you drive, so try to focus your thoughts on the exact present moment and the sensation of driving along.

How to Use Mindfulness

When you acquire the ability to sit and hone your thoughts onto the present moment only, you have achieved mindfulness. But what can you do with it? For one thing, you can use mindfulness to control how you think. When you notice that you are becoming negative and bitter, that you are dwelling on the past, or that you are worrying too much about the future, you can use mindfulness to draw your mind away from these depressing thoughts and making yourself focus on the present moment and whatever you are currently doing instead. You can also use mindfulness to become more aware and engaged with your present tasks, so that you do a better job and gain more confidence because of your good work. Finally, you can use mindfulness to gain appreciation for the present moment and all the wonderful things that life offers.

Chapter 4: Neuro-Linguistic Programming

Neuro-linguistic programming, hereafter referred to as NLP, is a great therapeutic technique designed for self-healing. By using NLP, you reprogram your mind and banish unwanted mental processes. You can become the person you want to be and gain more control over yourself.

NLP employs a variety of methods to help you change your thinking and your outlook on life. Visualization is one of the most common strategies that NLP uses. The therapy method teaches you to visualize your thoughts as material objects. By manipulating the visualizations, you can thus influence what you think and consequently you change how you feel. You can get rid of depression, anxiety, bad lifestyle habits such as smoking, and lack of motivation, among many things.

NLP also teaches you to change how you speak to affect how you and others think. By speaking in a more positive way, you encourage yourself to think more positively. Your mind is dramatically affected by what it hears, so if you hear yourself using more positive phrases, you will start thinking more positively.

Finally, NLP lets you reframe your life experiences. You can effectively alter how you look at life and how you feel about things with NLP reframing.

Visualizations

You can use visualizations to change how you process certain events in your life. Usually, if something upsets you, it seems huge and catastrophic to you. It will fill your mind as you assign it more and more importance. There is no need to give terrible things such importance. You can change this and make terrible things seem smaller to you by literally shrinking them down in size in your mind. Imagine that the thing that causes you so much angst is a snapshot in a picture frame. Now imagine that picture shrinking and shrinking until it fades out of your view. It is now so miniscule that you can't even see it, so it can't bother you anymore.

You can also imagine your fears, bad habits, toxic loved ones, or haunting past events as giant monsters. These monsters are ugly and scary, but you have a secret weapon. It is a special sword in your mind. You can either slay the monster, or else cut the monster down to a laughably small size. Either way, you should visualize using your own power to reduce each monster that terrorizes you into something small and harmless.

If you keep imagining the terrible or threatening words that someone said to hurt you, you can make their words seem less terrible by imagining them speaking to you in a cartoon voice. This removes the seriousness from what they are saying. It makes their words seem silly and inconsequential rather than hurtful. In the future, when this person speaks to you, just put a silly voice over his or her real voice. Get a good laugh, instead of another emotional wound.

When you want to feel more joy, peace, satisfaction, or happiness, then you can visualize the emotion that you want to feel as a color. Many people associate red with happiness, for instance, so imagine that happiness is the color red. Now imagine that you are drenching yourself in this color. This color is pervading you, filling every one of your cells. You become entirely red. Bathe yourself in the red color to make yourself happier every time.

Speech

Your choice in words, your tone, and your nonverbal body language all influences how others perceive your communication and how you perceive yourself. If you are saying nice things but your movements and tone imply that you are angry, then people will assume that you don't mean the nice things that you are saying. If you are lying and your body language and speech do not match up, people may suspect that you are lying. If you are constantly negative and pessimistic in your speech, then other people will find you to be a negative person and you will also bring yourself down.

The way that you speak can really impact the way that you think. If you choose to use more positive wording and words with more positive meanings, you will probably enjoy a more positive attitude. The way that you speak to yourself inside your head and the way that you speak to others out loud is very important. Make sure to be as positive and kind as possible in your internal and external speech.

For instance, choose to use action words, rather than passive words. This makes you feel more motivated and powerful. You can also choose to use more upbeat language. Instead of saying something like, "I have to go to my stupid job tomorrow," say, "I get to make money tomorrow!" Pick more positive words, too. Replace all negative words with words that have more positive connotations. Use a confident, upbeat tone to convey that you are confident and happy. Even if you are not actually confident and happy, you can make yourself feel that way by speaking in such a tone. Other people will respond to you better, and you will enjoy hearing yourself talk. Therefore, you will begin to feel better and think better.

In addition, you can really repair your relationships by improving your communication skills. Most relationships that you have with other people are actually quite fluid. You can repair damage done and change someone's opinion of you. You can do all of this just through communication. By being more direct, sympathetic, and positive in your speech, you can encourage other people to like you more. You can also avoid misunderstandings.

The main thing that you should do to improve your communication is to project more confidence, even if your confidence is fake. People will like and respect you more if you speak in a firm, unwavering voice and avoid phrases like "like," "um," and "well," as well as other filler words. Speaking with resolve communicates that you know what you are talking about and that you are sure of yourself and the situation. People like that and will feel more secure around you.

To forge better connections with people and end feelings of alienation and social isolation, you can dramatically improve your rapport by using two tricks known as mirroring and matching. Mirroring is where you mirror another person's movements and expressions. If someone cups his face in his hands and leans forward during conversation, for instance, you should copy his movements. Since people imitate the ones that they find attractive or agreeable, you will make people feel that you like them. By matching, you attempt to match your breathing rate to someone else's. This makes people subconsciously feel drawn to you and it creates a sense of trust.

Reframing

When something upsets you, you are really just choosing to be upset. You can reframe the events in your mind to calm down your emotions. Reframing is as simple as changing how you view a situation. Usually every situation and human interaction has several different interpretations. You can choose to use the worst interpretation possible, or you can choose one that hurts you less. It is always better to choose to think of situations in more positive lights, so try to choose the most positive framing possible.

Use reframing to change how you look at situations. Always ask yourself, "Are there things that I am missing? Am I focusing on the negative? How can I see the bright side in this situation?" Also consider that you do not have all of the information necessary to draw conclusion about something or someone, so reserve judgment.

Chapter 5: Self-Hypnosis

Self-hypnosis is a powerful therapeutic method that you can use on yourself to influence your thinking. It allows you to delve deep into your consciousness and plant helpful ideas there. It also allows you to find and address the causes of your emotional pain, if you are not sure why you feel the way that you do. While hypnosis can be performed by others, you can take full control of yourself and the hypnotic experience by performing it on yourself.

This form of self-therapy is useful for anyone. You can use it to induce relaxation and better stress reactions. You can suggest to your mind to stop thinking negatively, or to stop worrying and ruminating on things so much. You can even suggest to yourself that you drop certain unhealthy habits, such as smoking. Use self-hypnosis to alleviate pain, mental illness, bad habits, and lack of motivation.

How to Hypnotize Yourself

The key to hypnosis is reaching an impressionable state. During wakefulness, your subconscious is safely locked away from your conscious. However, during a hypnotic state, there is no barrier and your subconscious is easy to access. When you are in a hypnotic state, you can communicate openly with your subconscious. You can plant ideas and suggestions that your subconscious mind will receive and act on. Then, when you are conscious again, your subconscious will influence your conscious mind to think and act certain ways.

You can put yourself into a hypnotic state. First, you need to be in a quiet place where you will not be disturbed. All distractions, including music and cell phones, should be turned off. Sit in peace for a moment. Draw your attention to your breath; inhale and exhale, counting each breath. Now, focus on relaxing every part of your body. Find a spot on the wall to focus on as you calm each muscle. When you feel totally relaxed, tell yourself that you are bringing yourself back to awareness of your surroundings at the count of five. Then count from one to five. At five, sit upright and tense your muscles, while taking in the details of the room around you. Now, start relaxing again, and bring yourself back at the count of five. Repeat this whole process four or five times. Each time you relax, you will find that you relax a little more. You may also start to feel hazy or drowsy when you return to full consciousness. That is OK. The drowsiness just means that you are finally reaching your hypnotic state.

You can also use guided self-hypnosis tapes, CDs, or MP3s, which are available online. You can purchase or download guided hypnosis meditations for free. Use these guided meditations to help yourself relax and enter the hypnotic state.

When you become comfortable with accessing this hypnotic state, start to train yourself to respond to a cue. It could be the ringing of a bell or the sound of striking a meditation gong. Train yourself to enter your hypnotic state at the sound of this cue by playing the cue and then breathing and relaxing until you are in your hypnotic state. Soon, your mind will associate the cue with your hypnotic state and you will automatically slip into the state at the presence of the cue.

This is just preliminary training. It is supposed to help you learn what the hypnotic state feels like. It is also supposed to train your mind to become more receptive to hypnosis. Once you feel comfortable accessing the hypnotic state, you can begin to use self-hypnosis to achieve your goals.

Goals

You should create a clear and definite goal for yourself each time that you use hypnosis on yourself. Your goal should be something achievable and useful, such as becoming less depressed. Do away with vagueness and make sure that your goal is specific. Your subconscious won't be able to understand vague suggestions, only direct ones. It is OK to phrase your suggestion as an order, for your mind will respond to and obey any orders that it receives in the hypnotic state. Also make sure that your suggestions are in the present tense, so that your mind views them as a present goal that it can work on currently. Try to be positive and avoid terms like, "don't." Your subconscious will not listen to suggestions like, "Don't think so negatively anymore." Instead, it will just hear "think negatively." Try to use positive phrasing, such as, "Think more positively."

Now, when you are in a hypnotic state,

think of your goal. Suggest to yourself out loud

what you want to accomplish. "I want to wake up

at five in the morning," is one goal that you could

speak into your subconscious. "I will think

positively," is another goal.

Chapter 6: Schema-Focused Therapy

Schema-focused therapy is a fascinating form of therapy that targets on your schemas, or the way you see yourself. You can recreate your schema, or self-image, to be something that is healthy and wholesome. By doing this, you can change unhealthy and toxic patterns of thinking and behavior that you engage in. Your mind will thus make your personality and mental health fall into line to fit a better image. You will stop viewing yourself as a broken mess and instead you will view yourself as a positive being and you will love yourself more.

Usually, schema-based therapy is facilitated by a trained therapist. But you can use it on yourself with remarkable success. This therapy allows you to pinpoint and address negative thought patterns that you have fallen into the habit of thinking. When you think along these patterns, you can realize that you are hurting yourself and you can reframe the belief, or schema, to be something different.

Different Kinds of Schemas

Throughout your life, you form certain schemas, or beliefs. Most of your schemas formed early in childhood, but some of your schemas may have formed in adulthood. Your schemas shape your reality. They offer you a form of coping and a form of definition. Therefore, you cling to them like a life raft. Unfortunately, schemas are not always helpful. They may influence you to shape an unhealthy reality based on a negative and inaccurate image that you hold of yourself. Schemas are often maladaptive, meaning that you rely on them to help you but they are often unhelpful.

Because you rely on your schemas, you practice many behaviors to protect your self-beliefs. You don't like to let schemas go. You practice schema maintenance, where you selectively pick out and frame evidence from your life to support your schemas. For instance, if you think that you are fat and that no one can love you because of your weight, you use every form of rejection in your life as evidence that your weight makes you undesirable. Even if a rejection that you experience has nothing to do with your weight, you choose to believe that it does. You may also practice schema avoidance, where you repress your schemas because they cause you great discomfort. For instance, you might believe that you are unlovable because you have a terrible temper, so you become extremely sensitive to evidence that you have a bad temper and you avoid anything that makes you question the righteousness and necessity of your anger reactions. Finally, you may practice schema compensation, where you do the opposite of what your schemas suggest. You may secretly feel like a failure in life, so you overcompensate by aggressively and even obsessively fighting for success in all areas of your life. You may be a perfectionist to cover up your secret sense of failure and lack of control over life.

Part of schema therapy involves identifying your schemas. Identification calls for brutal honesty with yourself. You will have to recognize and address all of your schemas, including the uncomfortable ones that you try to repress through schema avoidance. In addition, you have to identify when you are practicing any sort of behavior to justify and protect your schemas, whether this behavior falls under the avoidance, compensation, or maintenance categories.

There are many schemas that you have. But here are some of the most common harmful ones:

- **Abandonment** – You secretly fear abandonment. You may have lost someone important to you in the past, so now you hold the belief that you will always be abandoned and let down by others. You approach your relationships with fear, because in your heart you think that no one that you love will be able to continue reliably providing you with emotional support or any other kind of support.

- **Mistrust -** You may believe that everyone is out to get you. You constantly fear that others have bad intentions and that your loved ones are secretly just out to hurt you. When you become emotionally involved with others, you watch them for signs that they are somehow manipulating, deceiving, or abusing you.

- **Emotional Deprivation** – You are constantly afraid that others will never be able to meet your emotional needs. There are three forms of deprivation that you may fear: a Deprivation of Nurturance, or the deprivation of warmth and affection; the Deprivation of Empathy, or the absence of sharing and warmth between people; or the Deprivation of Protection, or the lack of strength and protection by others.

- **Shame** – You are constantly ashamed of yourself. Somewhere inside your heart, you believe that you are inadequate and unlovable to others because you are somehow defective. You worry that people will stop loving you once you reveal who you truly are. Because you feel so flawed, you may have low self-esteem and you may be hyper sensitive to criticism or rejection of any kind.

- **Alienation** – You feel that you are alienated from the rest of the world and that you are too different from others to belong to any group or community.

- **Incompetence** – You are the unfortunate victim of a schema that makes you think that you are incapable of completing even simple living tasks on your own. As a result, you feel helpless and you rely on others too much. Living life on your own terrifies you.

- **Vulnerability to Harm or Illness** – You are constantly terrified that something bad will strike you at any time. You fear medical emergencies, environmental catastrophes, car accidents, plane crashes, or losing your job. Your life is basically a constant sense of dread and fear and worry.

- **Enmeshment/Undeveloped Self** – You fall prey to the belief that you are unable to survive without the full emotional support of another person, usually a significant other or one of your parents. You believe that you cannot survive without this other person and you fail to be independent. You may stay in abusive relationships as a result of your sense of co-dependency and enmeshment.

- **Failure** – You believe that you are destined to fail in every aspect of life. You also feel woefully inadequate compared to others and you do not believe in yourself. When you undertake a new activity or task, you find yourself expecting failure. Fear of failure may cause you to avoid or neglect many great opportunities in life.

- **Entitlement/Grandiosity -** Somehow you have developed a superiority complex. You believe that you are entitled to things and that you should be allowed to do whatever you want without consequences. You lack regard for the thoughts and feelings of others and you are entirely focused on what you deserve. You often feel like you are being discriminated against when you are not allowed special privileges; being told no is very hard for you to handle.

- **Insufficient Self-Control -** You do not take healthy control of your life. You follow your impulses and don't believe that you can control these impulses. As a result, your life is unstable and you have no control over your actions or emotions. You may also avoid responsibility and run away from commitment of any kind.

- **Subjugation** – You surrender your power to others and rely on others too much because you are too afraid to stand up for yourself. You do not feel like you are in control and you fear punishment if you do not surrender to others. Avoiding confrontation, abandonment, or anger is almost an obsession to you. There are two forms of subjugation that you may allow. You may surrender your needs, or you may suppress your emotions and pretend like everything is fine all of the time. Your emotions build up inside of you until one day you explode.

- **Self-Sacrifice** – Pleasing others is so important to you that you often overlook or sacrifice your own needs. You seek to gratify others at your expense. You are probably co-dependent and you do not stand up for yourself enough. The idea of asking for your needs to be met fills you with fear.

- **Approval-Seeking** – The approval of others is of paramount importance to you. You seek the approval of others constantly. You may even do things that you do not want to do, just to gain a head nod from other people. The approval of others makes you feel complete and balms your sense of inadequacy.

- **Pessimism** – You believe that the worst in life can and probably will happen. You fixate on the negative constantly and fear focusing on the positive too much. Your attitude brings you down, as well as others.

- **Emotional Inhibition** – You lock up your emotions and repress them in an attempt to please others or avoid losing control of yourself. You are constantly bottled up. You may also avoid saying no when you should.

- **Hypercriticalness** – You set ridiculously high and unreasonable standards of perfection for yourself. When you fail to meet these unrealistic expectations, you feel like a failure and you criticize yourself for everything. You also have an inflated sense of responsibility and blame yourself for things that are beyond your control. The world rests on your shoulders and you feel like it will burn if you do not do everything that you can to be perfect.

- **Punitiveness** – You believe that people must be harshly punished for everything that they do wrong. You are overly critical, intolerant, and harsh. You lack empathy and compassion and do not allow for imperfection or human error.

Three Steps

Schema therapy involves three crucial steps. The first is the assessment phase. The second is awareness, where you gain an understanding of what your schemas look like and you learn to spot them in your daily life. The final phase is the replacement phase, where you work on replacing your negative schemas with more positive ones.

Assessment

You can use a questionnaire downloaded from the Internet to help find out what your schemas are. You can also use personal introspection. Which of the above schemas seem to describe you? Don't be afraid to start a journal, where you explore the schemas that seem to dictate your life and define who you are. You need to be brutally honest with yourself, even if it hurts. This phase may be uncomfortable and even overwhelming, but it is the shortest phase of the therapeutic process. After it is over, you will feel better.

Awareness

Start noticing when one of your schemas acts up. Do you avoid opportunities because you fear that you will fail? Do you watch your spouse closely for signs of cheating, to the point where you imagine evidence that he or she is unfaithful? Notice how and when your schemas cause you to behave in certain ways. Gaining this awareness will motivate you to change and will help you identify when you need to replace a negative pattern with a positive one.

Replacement

Once you know what your schemas are and how they affect your human experience, start to analyze them. Find beliefs that are more positive and beneficial. For instance, if you are punitive and intolerant of others, start trying to forgive others for their small errors and excuse human imperfections and flaws. Remember that you are not perfect but you would like mercy, right? If you are hyper critical of yourself, remind yourself that you are not perfect and the world will not stop spinning if you do not do everything. Wherever you hold a negative belief, find a more positive one.

Now, when you notice that you are thinking along one of your negative patterns, you can change it. Replace the negative thoughts that you think based on your schemas with more positive thoughts. You will notice that your life begins to change and become more positive.

Chapter 7: Metaphysical

Metaphysical self-healing uses the belief in your own energy as a means to healing your mind, body, and spirit. Metaphysical healing focuses more on spiritual healing, light energy, and clearing away negative energy. Whether or not you believe in spirituality, viewing your pain as negative energy and your potential happiness as positive energy or light is a powerful form of symbolism that you can use to train your mind to heal itself. This form of self-healing can create an excellent and powerful mental picture that can help your mind let go of pain and accept happiness.

If you do believe in energy and spirituality, you can use this method to balance your energy and feel better as a spiritual being. You will find great power in using spiritual methods for ascending above the pain that negative energy and negative thinking causes you.

Ascension

I have already introduced the idea that you are more powerful than you realize. However, ascension healing takes this idea a step further by teaching the concept that you are a conduit for spiritual energy and that you hold the keys to your own healing in your spiritual makeup. You can channel the energy that you need to heal, if you so choose. Everyone has a healing power within them. You just have to hone yours and concentrate it on yourself and your wounds. You must channel positive energy, love, and healing light, instead of the more negative energy that keeps your wounds open.

The reasons ascension healing works is because it elevates your spiritual energy. You become higher in your vibrational energy. You take your spiritual power and healing into your own hands, which boosts your confidence and gives you much-needed control over your own life. You can essentially ascend your emotional pain, mental illness, and other problems by increasing and improving the quality of the energy that you allow into your spirit. By only allowing positive energy and light into your existence, you become a stronger and spiritually healthier person. Thus, you feel better and you are able to heal. You no longer allow negative forces to hinder you and lower your energy, making you feel bad.

A lot of the negativity in your life is self-generated. This may seem harsh, but if you think about it, your pain is often caused by your poor thinking patterns and general sense of despair, anger, unhappiness, and/or hopelessness. By embracing positive energy, you become happier. You stop letting yourself build up negative energy within by thinking in unhelpful ways and harboring negative emotions. When a negative thought or emotion begins to bother you, you can visualize bathing your inner self with loving white light. This visualization will help dispel the negative energy generated by your thought or emotion, and will fill you with joy instead.

Sometimes, life will throw negative people or circumstances at you. You are not responsible for every negative thing that you are exposed to, but you are responsible for how you handle this negativity. When you are using ascension healing, you should elevate yourself above the negativity of life events that are beyond your control. When negative things happen to you or you are forced to be around negative people, the bad energy can drain you of all happiness and joy. It can ruin your peace, as well. Imagine yourself rising above it and purifying yourself from the toxic effects of the negative event by washing yourself in healing light.

In addition to healing yourself with positive energy, you must embrace a more positive lifestyle. You should choose to surround yourself with positivity as much as possible. Kick out the negative things and events that you can. Try to live a good, pure life that you are happy with. Keeping a positive mindset and smiling will do wonders to elevate your vibrational energy, helping you skim along above the negative forces that try to pull you down into a mire of hurt and chaos.

The positive white light that you bathe yourself in is a powerful metaphor for positive energy and life forces. You do not have to believe in energetic healing to gain benefit from imagining loving white light that heals all of your emotional wounds and repairs your life. This visualization will simply encourage your mind to stay positive and take care of itself despite the bumps and bruises that are inevitable in life.

Your spirituality is not something that you should neglect. Rather, you should embrace your spirituality and take care of it. Take care of yourself.

Another great thing about ascension healing is that you are treating yourself as a whole being. You are healing your mind, body, and spirit all at once. Since every part of you works together to create a unified whole, this holistic approach is very helpful. It allows you to address all of your problems and heal yourself completely.

Four Agreements

The Four Agreements are four cardinal rules for you to follow. These Agreements are based on Toltec wisdom taught by Don Miguel

Ruiz. Basically, you want to apply these Agreements to all areas of your life in order to achieve spiritual, mental, and even physical peace and happiness. These Agreements must become habitual to work. Though you are sure to lapse at first, eventually you will find it easy to follow these Agreements and enjoy the benefits that they offer.

You should try to apply this wisdom to your life every day. Use it to heal your mind, body, and spirit by taking care of yourself and leading a life that is free of strife. Use it to gain control over yourself and achieve the peace and healing that you need to feel well.

The first Agreement is to be impeccable with your word. You must speak with integrity and do what you say that you will do. You must avoid doing things like lying or manipulating people, as these actions are not impeccable and will lower the strength of your vibrational energy. You will feel guilty and invite negative repercussions for your negative behavior. Instead of behaving in ways that are not admirable or impeccable, you should strive to be a good person. In the end, you will reap great rewards and your life will be better.

The second is to avoid taking things personally. Not everything in life is about you. By not taking things so personally, you will reduce a lot of your pain. You will have more energy to dedicate to your spiritual health and wellness. Stop worrying about what other people think of you; their thoughts are none of your business. Stop thinking that people are unhappy with you just because they act rudely or coldly toward you; the way that they treat you is because of their own issues, not any flaws in your being. Stop assuming that people are talking about you or judging you; most people are so focused on themselves that they barely notice you at all anyway. Your energy and your health is your business, so focus on that. The actions, words, and attitude of others are not actually part of your life, so don't let it consume you.

The third is to stop making assumptions. You may have heard the saying that when you assume, you make an ass of you and me. Assumptions are likely a huge cause of your unhappiness and mental strife. How often do you assume that someone hates you because he or she did not return your calls? You work yourself up into a state of anxiety and misery thinking that someone hates you, then you find out that the person was just busy or dealing with some sort of problem and did not have time to return your calls. Or perhaps you assumed that someone was angry with you based on something that you did. You later find out that the person was not really angry at all. You dedicate a lot of emotional energy and inflict a lot of pain on yourself by making assumptions. It is better to never assume and to find things out for yourself.

The fourth is to always strive to do your very best in all areas of your life. Trying your best makes you feel good. You know that you tried, even if you fail. You also raised your vibrational energy and feel better because you are driven by your will to do a good job in all areas of life.

People will see how much you try, and they will respect your efforts. The harder you try, the better you will do in life. You will start to enjoy more confidence and more success in life as you begin doing your best. When you lag in energy and do things poorly, you actually pit yourself against your own well-being and drag yourself down. Avoid doing this by always trying your best at everything that you do.

Integrating these Four Agreements into your life will help you heal yourself because you will grow your confidence and reduce the things that cause you pain. You will fix your lifestyle habits to be more healthy and conducive to your success.

On top of integrating these Four Agreements in your daily life, you must start to work on cutting out bad habits. Doing things that hurt your success and forward progress in life is the opposite of self-healing. Using Toltec wisdom and the Four Agreements to heal yourself calls for you to ditch bad habits and embrace healthy ones.

Restorative Touch

Restorative touch is related to reiki. This is a form of spiritual healing that encourages you to utilize your own natural healing energy to heal yourself. You can begin the healing process by touching yourself and channeling loving energy through your fingers. The way that you touch different parts of your body can help you feel better and can help you heal yourself. Using loving and restorative touch is supposed to help you foster self-love and caring for yourself.

There is no right or wrong way to use restorative touch. As long as you are touching yourself with love, you will help heal yourself. Touch yourself over the chest to mend your broken heart, over the temples to quiet your anxious mind, and over your throat to heal your sense of inadequacy or not being heard and appreciated by others.

Meditation

Meditation is an important act of self-love and self-healing. Taking some quiet time to reflect on your life and to get in touch with your inner voice, or spiritual voice, is essential for your overall peace and happiness. It has been found that people who meditate are generally happier and possess a greater sense of peace and direction in life. This is because people who routinely meditate take the time to quiet the distractions in their lives and get in touch with their spirit. They bother to listen to themselves and let their spirit guide them through the mayhem in life that so often feels hopelessly confusing.

Meditation does not have to be extremely spiritual. However, your purpose in meditation should be to quiet your mind's chatter so that you can access the wisdom that you already possess deep in your spirit. You are essentially tuning out all distractions to hear what your inner self really has to say. If you are religious, you may use meditation to access the information that a higher power will try to impart to you without the distraction and clutter of outside stimulus.

You must take some time to meditate without distraction. Turn off music, cell phones, computers, and other forms of stimulus. Sit in quiet reflection for a while. Use breathing to ground yourself and quiet your mind. Do not let your mind wander onto thoughts; instead, stay focused on the present moment. You may choose to pray or to use a guided meditation that directs you along a path of visualizations to reach some sort of conclusion. You may also just choose to sit in Zen peace. It is up to you how you choose to meditate. There is no right or wrong way. What works for you best is how you should approach meditation. If you have no idea where to begin, experiment with a few different kinds of meditation to find what works best for you.

Prayer

Religious people swear by the power of prayer. Prayer can certainly ground you in your religious conviction, connect you to your chosen deity, and help you feel wholesome again. You can use prayer to help facilitate self-healing.

Regardless of your religion, prayer and spiritual meditation are probably a large part of the rituals in your worship. This is because prayer is incredibly powerful for your spiritual health. By praying to your deity and meditating on religious things, you can begin to mend your spirit. You stop feeling so alone, as you connect with your spiritual beliefs and honor your religious convictions. In addition, you entrust your burdens to a higher power, which helps release you of some of the stress that you choose to carry on your shoulders. You really can survive without that stress. Most of the things that you worry about are beyond your control. Trust them to your higher power, and free yourself to focus on the important things in life that you can control.

It is often helpful to seek counsel from a clergy member or other religious figure in your spiritual community. This figure can help you feel closer to your deity or deities. He or she can also offer you advice to gaining inner peace and spiritual freedom and purity. You will find that you feel better after speaking to someone in your religious community. Religious figures can be as soothing and helpful as expensive therapists.

Just taking some time for worship and prayer is an act of self-love, as well. You take some time to do something positive and meaningful to you. You take a break from the stresses and cares of everyday life, in order to focus on what matters to your spirit. Take some time out of your hectic schedule to pray and connect with your religion.

Conclusion

Hopefully by now you are feeling both prepared and excited for the commencement of your self-healing journey. After reading this book, you are now aware that self-healing is not only possible, but extremely beneficial and necessary to your overall health and happiness. There are countless ways to begin self-healing, but the power to heal yourself lies within you. Some of the most successful and popular techniques have been discussed here. Therefore, you should now be ready to start your journey of self-healing.

Self-healing will not be easy. In fact, it will be a wild ride. Sometimes you will backslide or even fail your goals. But instead of hating

yourself, you should just keep moving forward.
Keep trying. Never give up. Self-healing is a
process and often it does not move in a linear
fashion. Rather, your progress will zigzag. That
does not mean that you are not healing. You are
healing, and you just need to be patient with
yourself and treat yourself with love.

Self-love is the cornerstone of self-
healing. You cannot reasonably expect yourself
to heal from your emotional and mental wounds
if you are always beating yourself up. Be kind to
yourself and treat yourself as you would a best
friend whom you deeply love. Your attitude will
help facilitate your healing.

Your attitude should also be positive.
Negative thoughts and actions only add to your
pain and cripple the self-healing process. By

being positive, you open yourself up for healing. You allow the goodness that healing brings to infiltrate your life and fill your inner self with energy. Suddenly, you will feel better and you will feel motivated to achieve your goals and dreams. By moving forward on your goals and dreams, you distract yourself from the pain of the past and you suddenly find yourself able to let go of negative self-beliefs. Your wounds will no longer be fostered by an environment of negativity and mental paralysis. Your self-esteem will no longer suffer and you will no longer hate yourself because you are too negative and stuck in the pain of the past to move on with what you want in life.

Once you start loving yourself and being positive, you will be able to heal. But sometimes loving yourself and being positive is difficult if you are used to more negative patterns. Therefore, consider this all part of the healing process. Work on it each day, but don't beat yourself when you slide back in progress. You are doing better than you think. You are trying to heal yourself without therapy or medication, which is an amazing and admirable feat.

Open yourself up to a great future. Your future is yours, so make it what you want it to be. No matter what has happened to you or how you have acted in the past, you have the opportunity for a great future. You can heal yourself and move forward instead of staying stuck in the same rut in life. You can finally feel happy and content, and achieve your dreams, regardless of what mental illnesses you suffer or what terrible

past events you have endured.